6 Weeks of Anywhere HIIT Workouts for Women

Quick, effective results that tone & strengthen, for home or travel, scaled at three levels to meet your current fitness & equipment needs

Elisa Pool

CONTENTS

INTRODUCTION

Welcome! My name is Elisa Pool and I've created this resource for women everywhere who want quick, effective workouts that they can do anywhere they find themselves – whether that be at home, in the garage, or on the road. Why? Because while I love going to a gym to work out, I don't always have the time to make that happen. And that's coming from a previous gym owner!

As a mom of two kids and the caretaker for my mom, I don't always have time to drive to the gym, do the workout, and then drive back. After all, there is dinner to make, activities to chauffeur kids to and from, laundry to do, and, of course, work to get done!

So, this collection of workouts is designed to help YOU, the busy woman, get a great workout that will strengthen your body, boost your mood, and elevate your fitness – even if you don't have much space, equipment, or time. And, if you're worried about your fitness level, put your mind at ease. Every single workout has three levels, so you can decide which level suits you best each day.

I have personally done every single one of these workouts, some of them many times! They are fast, simple and effective. I'm going to explain everything so you feel confident and motivated.

Let's get you going!

1

TYPES OF EXERCISE AND BENEFITS

We all know that exercise is important. But do you know HOW important? Exercise has been shown over and over (and OVER) again to:

- Improve mood

- Decrease depression

- Increase bone density

- Improve heart health

- Enhance circulation & respiratory ability

- Help us lead longer lives

- Improve our sleep

- Lower our stress levels

- Calm us down

- Lower inflammation

- Protect our brain against cognitive decline and brain shrinkage

- Keep our brain younger

After hearing that list, I ask you, why would anyone NOT want to exercise?

Dr. Lisa Mosconi, author of The XX Brain, explains that, "Exercise causes actual physical changes in the brain that not only act as a safeguard against future dementia, but also invigorate our abilities to think, reason, and remember."

My grandmother had severe Alzheimer's disease, so I am *all* about healthy brain function, and this is huge for me. I would guess it's important to you, also, because how much can we really enjoy life if our brains don't work well?

Exercise also stimulates the production of growth hormone and brain-derived neurotrophic factor (BDNF), which promotes our neurons' abilities to build new connections. It also acts as a repair kit for any slightly damaged brain cells. This leads to increased plasticity and connectivity, improving our ability to make and retain memories. Another important brain activity: remembering!

Exercise keeps our DNA young - with evidence showing NINE fewer years of aging at the cellular level among people who exercise regularly. The bottom line is, Dr. Mosconi believes that exercise is as critical to women's health as mammograms and annual checkups!

So let's get technical. What is this exercise we need?

Exercise can be defined as "intentionally planned, structured, repetitive movement intended to improve or maintain physical fitness."

Usually, people think of exercise as activities like going to the gym, CrossFit, treadmills, playing tennis, sports, bicycling, jumping, weight lifting, karate, swimming, etc. Walking 5,000 to 10,000 steps a day is also a basic exercise that most people can achieve with focused effort.

There are numerous *ways* to exercise, but there are three major *types* of exercise that are hugely beneficial to incorporate into your life, which I will briefly summarize here: cardiovascular exercise, strength training, and high intensity interval training.

Just like our bodies do better with a variety of foods (instead of eating the same kinds of foods over and over), our bodies do better with a variety of exercise types (instead of doing the same exercise over and over).

Why is that? It's because our bodies have different metabolic pathways, and each kind of exercise stimulates different pathways, and have different benefits!

Strength Training

Strength training, also known as resistance training, helps you build and maintain that vital muscle mass we want (you'll learn more about that in the next chapter), which is *especially* critical as we age. Strength training several times a week is one of the best things you can do for your health, especially for women, because in addition to the benefits of building muscle, it will boost your confidence, sex drive, and overall mood.

Strength training has also been shown to slow down amyloid plaques - which are the things that accumulate in people with dementia and Alzheimers. As of 2022, Alzheimers was the 7th leading cause of death in the USA, and is continually increasing - so the fact that strength training can stall the acceleration of those amyloid plaques is powerful!

No matter what your current ability or age, the goal is to start incorporating resistance or strength training 2-3x a week minimum. What this could look like is using resistance bands, resistance machines, free weights like dumbbells or barbells, or kettlebells. It can even look like using your own body, in compound movements like push ups, squats, and pull ups! Compound movements use multiple muscle groups and offer plentiful muscle building benefits.

Isolated movements (like bicep curls or calf raises) can also help, starting with sets in the range of 8-12 reps of a heavier weight for a few weeks, then vary it up with sets of higher reps, like 20-30, using a slightly lighter weight. The goal with strength training is to move your body in sets of movements with a weight that whatever you are doing starts to feel HARD – as in it takes *real* effort to complete it towards the end of your rep counts – so don't be afraid to try the heavier weights!

Cardiovascular Exercise

Cardiovascular exercise, or what people often refer to as "cardio," improves the health of your cardiovascular system and respiratory endurance, strengthens the heart, burns calories, and can improve your recovery. Cardiovascular exercise usually consists of monostructural movements that involve a single, repetitive motion that can be repeated for extended periods of time. Examples include running, hiking, rowing, biking, swimming, and jump rope. Monostructural movements are low-skill and highly practical because most people can find one they like.

Walking is a great example of cardiovascular exercise we can all do. Don't underestimate it! Humans were made for walking (just look at how we stand on two feet as an example), and brisk walking is one of the biggest indicators of longevity.

High Intensity Interval Training

High Intensity Interval Training (HIIT) are highly efficient workouts that are short (usually between 15-30 minutes), but intense, making them ideal for people with busy schedules. As a bonus, they have multiple benefits.

For example, HIIT improves your body's handling of blood sugar, improves your cardiovascular health by alternating periods of intense exercise and recovery, and increases your muscle mass.

Significantly, HIIT boosts your metabolism and helps you burn fat more efficiently. How?

There's this phenomenon called EPOC (excess post-exercise oxygen consumption), which means that your body burns more calories, even *hours* after the workout is finished. I'm guessing we can all agree that burning more calories after you've finished working out is a pretty great benefit, especially knowing that it also supports cardiovascular health, insulin sensitivity, and fat loss.

Regular HIIT training can increase your endurance capacity as well, both aerobic (endurance) and anaerobic (short bursts of power), improving your overall fitness and stamina.

HIIT and resistance training also improve your bone density, which is vital if you want to avoid osteoporosis and other skeletally degenerative issues. To remineralize the bones of your body, you need a weight load or some kind of impact to allow the calcium in the bones to become denser. No load or no impact means no pressure on the bones to get stronger.

Strength training and HIIT workouts typically require more focus and presence of mind than monostructural "cardio" movements. Depending on the movement, you might even be building new neurological pathways, which is excellent for your brain health. Your brain is also a muscle, so the more you use and challenge it, the better.

Putting It All Together

What makes the workouts in this book so effective is that most fall under the categories of High Intensity Interval Training and strength training.

All types of exercise have been shown to improve your overall mental and physical health, so ideally, you want all types! However, the most important type of exercise is the one you actually DO, so whatever that is, *do it!* It's too important not to exercise.

The goal is to move your body intentionally, at least a little, 4-6 days a week or more. A nice balance for the majority of middle-aged women is to mix 2-3 days a week of low to moderate intensity cardio or strength training with 2-3 days a week of higher intensity workouts that you find in this book. You'll find more suggestions to consider in chapter four, so check those out to see what might work best for you. I almost always recommend giving yourself at least one day a week of physical rest, regardless.

Remember, YOUR level of training is different from mine, and mine is different from an elite athlete. You start with where you are and build slowly.

2

BUILDING MUSCLE, NOT BULK

M uscles respond to the demands you put on them. If you ask your muscles to lift heavy things, they will start getting stronger. If you ask your muscles to sit on the couch, they will slowly start to shrivel away – and you get weaker along the way.

The way we build muscle is actually by damaging them. We cause small tears in the tissue, and then they repair themselves bigger and stronger. This is why resistance training or strength training is so helpful. It's a positive stress on our body.

"But what if I bulk up?"

This is a concern that I still hear frequently from women. (For your reference, there are two author pictures in the back of the book -one to show you what my muscle mass looks like while working out, and one to show you how it looks at rest.

An old neighbor once told me, "No offense, it looks great on you, but I don't want that for me." None taken, and my question is, WHY don't you want it for yourself? Muscle is, hands down, one of the most important tissues on our bodies. Here are seven reasons why:

1. **If you want to be TONE and slimmer** (which is what I hear from most women) **you get that from building muscle, not from losing fat.** Muscle radically affects your body composition, and the reason why you don't bulk up is because muscle takes up ¼ to ⅓ *less* space than fat. That means, if you convert some fat to muscle, even though you weigh more, your body will be tighter and more sculpted. You can weigh the same or *more* with lean muscle mass, but wear a different, *smaller*, size of clothing. I actually weigh more now than I did in college and I am two sizes smaller. (Side note: I dare you to google 5 lbs of muscle vs fat images.) It would require a LOT of time and strength building - more than three times a week - to build enough muscle to bulk up more than you were, since muscle is so dense.

2. **If you are trying to lose weight, muscle is especially important!** Many times when people lower their calorie consumption to lose weight, the body ends up using muscle tissue as energy and eating into your muscles instead of fat stores. You actually *lose* muscle, which then *slows down* your metabolism. Hear me now: a slower metabolism is NOT what you want when

you are trying to lose weight. The way to fight that is by building more muscle. Strength training will help you maintain your weight loss, because it's helping *build* muscles instead of losing them — which is what you want!

3. **Muscle mass improves your insulin sensitivity.** As you may or may not know, being sensitive to insulin is critical if you want to maintain good health long term. Insulin resistance (when your body is no longer sensitive to insulin) is a major proponent of numerous chronic health issues, such as type 2 diabetes, cardiovascular disease, obesity and even Alzheimers. Have you ever noticed that many people who are more muscular also have lower body fat? They usually have better insulin control, too. This is because muscle is one of the main places your body can absorb blood glucose (the sugar in your blood after eating). The more muscle you have, the more blood glucose it can absorb. If you don't have a lot of muscle, that capacity is filled quickly, so the rest of the blood sugar is stored as triglycerides in the fat cells (some blood glucose can be stored in the liver, but that is also a limited quantity).

4. **Muscles raise your Resting Metabolic Rate (RMR).** This means that the more lean muscle mass you have, the more calories you burn while you are doing absolutely nothing. Sounds nice, right? This is because muscle mass burns more calories! Muscles require energy (calories) to

contract and relax. Because muscles require so much energy to maintain, they burn more of the calories you eat simply by existing. This means even when you're not moving, muscle cells are burning calories. One pound of muscle burns more calories than one pound of fat. Why not build more muscle to help your metabolic function?

5. **Your muscle mass helps you as you age.** Often we associate aging with a loss of muscle mass, which is known as sarcopenia. Think of elderly people, and how uncommon it is to see muscle definition on them. It shouldn't come as surprise to learn that osteoporosis and bone fractures are more common as we age. By preserving muscle mass, we can preserve strength - which is a predictor of survival as a person ages. Which leads me to the next point:

6. **Your skeletal mass improves your overall body's capabilities.** Muscle affects your organs, tissues, immune system, and is a great biomarker for overall health. Generally speaking, larger muscles are stronger muscles, and this leads to improved movement and daily function in most people. As you build more muscle, you become more capable.

7. **Muscle is critical to your overall health.** Lean muscle mass has been shown to lower LDL cholesterol, as well as increase human growth hormone, which repairs tissue, bone, skin and main-

tains fat levels. Muscle is a reservoir for your amino acids, and is the most metabolically active tissue you have. Muscle also helps us survive if we have to fight off infectious diseases!

As you can see, building muscle mass is essential to your overall health. It is a huge benefit! I once had a trainer say that weight lifting was the fountain of youth, and after learning all of this, she may have been onto something!

3

PROTEIN'S PART

The first way to build muscles is by exercising. The second way to get more muscle mass is to eat more protein (which is a guideline I enjoy, because I like to eat!).

Protein is hugely important for both building and maintaining muscle mass. We must eat protein to promote muscle synthesis, which means we need to eat protein in order for our bodies to make muscle tissue... and keep it.

As you age, your skeletal muscle changes. Muscle actually becomes LESS efficient as we age (due to multiple factors like being more sedentary, having higher rates of illness, and others).

When you're young, you can get away with eating less protein. However, when you hit your 30s and 40s, your metabolic health will definitely benefit from you having a plan to consume more protein. Did you catch that age? Your 30s, ladies!! That's not even mid-life.

So, how much protein do we need to be eating? For people who want to improve metabolic function, lose weight, or hit a body composition goal, a healthy target is one gram of protein per pound of ideal body weight. So, if your goal is to weigh 150 pounds, for instance, you're aiming to eat 150 grams of protein a day.

Dr. Gabrielle Lyon, a board-certified family physician who is trained in geriatric nutritional sciences, says the two most important meals are the first meal of the day (whenever that is eaten), and the last meal of the day. In between isn't as critical.

The reason getting high amounts of protein in the first and last meals of the day is so important is because the amount of protein you eat can signal muscle protein synthesis. It's as if there were a switch in the body that when you eat a certain amount of protein at one time, the body turns on the "make muscle" function. How much protein is that? It's 40-50 grams of protein.

So, you might have 40g of protein at breakfast, 50g at dinner, and divvy up the rest during the day as you see fit.

To offer an idea of what that might look like, I'll share my typical protein intake for the day. Since my goal is maintaining my current muscle mass, on an average day, I eat:

Breakfast: Monday through Saturday, I eat three pasture-raised eggs with 2-3 servings of chopped and sauteed cruciferous vegetables, mixed with some ground turkey meat. I usually have a few berries, too, or some other kind of fruit. It's around 40-45g of protein.

Dinner: I eat two servings of the protein from the meal, more veggies (often in the form of field greens), and moderate carbs; also around 40-45g of protein.

Lunch: it's usually either leftovers from the day before, or a protein shake, but there's always protein in there somewhere, and if there isn't, I notice, because I get hungry!

Do I always eat ALL the protein I want each day? No, and that's okay. However, I am very intentional about getting a LOT of protein each day, and it makes a huge difference.

Protein (along with seeds & nuts) is my go-to if I want a snack or am feeling hungry. I'll grab some marinated chicken thighs I keep around, or have a half shake, or something along those lines. However, I've noticed that if I eat enough protein three times a day, I don't feel the need to snack very much, which is great!

If you are feeling hungry throughout the day, I encourage you to *eat more protein*, for a few reasons:

First, protein has a very high satiety rating - meaning it makes you feel full.

Second, studies show it is the best kind of calorie to consume if you are feeling hungry but trying to keep calorie count low. It's lower in calories than fats, and you burn more calories eating protein than you do carbs or fat. (Yes, different foods burn more calories when you eat them than others.)

Another interesting thing about eating protein is that it has been found to make girls less driven to eat sweet foods - which can be very helpful!

The bottom line is, you want to prioritize getting protein in your diet each day, multiple times a day. Mix and match protein sources to get the amount you need.

Where do you find protein?

Red meats like grass-fed beef, bison, and elk are packed with minerals your body needs and are excellent sources of protein. They are not carcinogenic or harmful in terms of cholesterol as we once thought.

Poultry, like chicken, turkey, duck or quail are also help-ful sources; wild-caught fish, shrimp and other seafood; pasture-raised eggs are also all great sources. (I am a huge proponent of eating meat from regenerative farms and / or wild-caught options. I know that's not always possible, but that is where we choose to invest as often as possible. The wilder the meat, typically that means the fewer additives / hormones/ antibiotics in the food of that animal, the higher nutrient profile, and a higher quality of life.)

You can also mix plant sources of protein, like quinoa, buckwheat, and amaranth, though you have to eat over 3 cups of quinoa to get the protein from one 4-ounce chicken breast, and that is a LOT of quinoa. If your goal is weight loss, you'll want to be aware of the quantity of those complex carbs you are eating.

One more thing you want to remember if you are eating protein from NON animal sources (as many of us do, including myself): Vegetable proteins are not complete proteins; meaning, they don't have all the amino acids necessary for protein synthesis. So, if your protein is typically plant-based, find out which amino acids you are consuming to figure out which other ones you need to add in to get that profile. Typically with plant-based foods, you need to mix and match two or three sources to get a mix of amino acids.

If you would like some ideas for high-protein, nutrient-dense meals, here are two resources for you. One of these QR codes will take you to 6 free high-protein breakfast ideas, and the other will take you to five Family Friendly Meal Ideas (some of our personal family favorites).

High Protein Breakfast Ideas

Five Family Friendly Meals

4

LEARN YOUR LEVEL

Each workout in this book offers three variations: "Keep Me Moving", "Kick It Up a Notch", and "Turbo Boost Me." Many people would look at these and see workouts for beginners, intermediate, and advanced, and that's certainly one way to look at them.

They are also designed with other things in mind, like different intensity levels, equipment on hand, or time allowed — and I encourage everyone to have a broader view of their wellness and fitness. As someone who could physically choose the "Turbo Boost Me" option each time I work out, I often choose one of the other two, or mix and match some of the movements, due to mood or location.

It's wise to have options for several reasons, outlined on the next few pages.

Menstruation Cycles

If you are still menstruating, your body is on a biological rhythm that lasts longer than the 3-5 days you actually are menstruating. Your hormones are fluctuating all month long, and go through several massive changes at other times in your life (puberty, pregnancy, and menopause). Exact experiences are unique to each woman, of course, but there are some generalities I can offer for your consideration.

The chart below summarizes what happens during the four phases of the Menstruation Cycle. Use it to gain a better understanding of what's happening internally, so that you can listen more closely to your body and adjust your food, sleep, and exercise as needed. Remember, this is an approximation, not an exact printout of your biology or what will work for you. On the days you want to go lighter, use the "Keep Me Moving" workouts. When you're feeling energized and ready to go, use the "Turbo Boost Me" options.

Note: *Avoid one-size-fits-all thinking!* You must experiment, and learn to pay attention to and listen to your body. In my personal experience, my ability to exercise does *not* follow this pattern every month. While most months I want to lay low the first two days of my period, there have been months where I have wanted to sprint during that time, or lift really heavy weights. Trust your body to tell you what it needs.

THE MENSTRUAL CYCLE			
STAGE	Menstruation (Follicular)	Follicular	Ovulatory	Luteal
DAYS	1-5	6-14	15-17	18-28
SUMM-ARY OF STAGE	Uterus lining sheds, creating blood	Preps to receive egg, releases luteinizing hormone (LH) and follicle stimulating hormones (FSH) to release eggs; one matures, others reabsorbed	Egg leaves the ovary and travels through tubes to uterus	Follicle becomes a Corpus Luteum and secretes progesterone. If egg isn't fertilized, the CL dissolves, estrogen & progesterone drop abruptly, PMS can develop
HOR-MONES	Estrogen and progesterone both low	Estrogen levels are low, but steadily increase - a balance between too much & too little estrogen; can fluctuate	Peaks in estrogen, progesterone and testosterone	Sudden drops in estrogen, FSH, LH, progesterone, higher blood glucose levels
EXPER-IENCE	Energy levels lower, and possibly mood	Slower metabolism, lower cortisol, higher energy levels, good moods	Higher sex drive, more confidence, higher energy levels	Hungrier as energy intake increases, more food cravings, lower energy levels, moodiness
EXER-CISE	Light, low movement, slow yoga, stretching, meditation, connecting with nature, walking	Cardio exercise, HIIT; hiking, running, jogging, heavier weights, cross-training	Sprinting, HIIT, running, spinning, circuit training, going for heavier weights at fewer reps, one rep maxes	Stamina may be low, so do light or moderate exercise for longer time periods, controlled strength training, pilates, yoga, walking

Age & Era

As previously mentioned, our female bodies go through major changes each day of the month, and over and over again throughout our lives.

Typically speaking, when we are young and our hormones are at their peak operating levels, we can hit our workouts hard, and it's in our benefit to do so (these gains stay with us for years to come). As we age, our hormones change, and we benefit from other intensity levels. Below are the eras of our lives and the levels that may most benefit us. Once again these are approximations and generalizations, so be sure to do your own thinking here as you consider your personal experience and conditioning level when implementing your own exercise routine.

Age & Era	Exercise Level	Types of Exercise
Ages 18-20 Childless Women	Turbo Boost Me Others as needed	High intensity 4-5x a week
Childbearing Women	Keep Me Moving Kick It Up a Notch	Mid to Low Intensity cardio Slow Strength Training
Ages 35-45 Perimenopause	Kick It Up a Notch Turbo Boost Me	2-3 days strength training, 2-3 days HIIT, Mid intensity cardio
Ages 50+ Post Menopause	Keep Me Moving Kick It Up a Notch Turbo Boost Me	2-3 days strength training, 2-3 days HIIT, Low intensity cardio for longer time

Injuries

Injury *can* happen in any sport, bottom line. Many injuries happen because of speed, overuse, not paying attention, or improper self care. Truth be told, I have had far *fewer* issues and injuries from HIIT and strength training than any other kind of exercise (like running). Perhaps the reason is because you are often moving in a more focused way.

The easiest way to avoid injury is to check your form and speed. Read the description for each movement, watch the demonstration videos provided and pay attention to your form. If you go too heavy, too fast, you could hurt yourself. If you pay attention and move slowly and deliberately, you should be fine. If you are concerned about a movement, speak with a doctor or simply don't do it.

If you are recently starting out after a longer period away from exercise, it's probably in your best interest to adjust more slowly than you think to a new workout regimen.

If you are in pain, *stop*. There's a way out of it. Work with an expert to find the issue sooner rather than later so that your body doesn't make a habit out of overcompensating, which usually creates other problems down the road.

Body Individualities

We all have our own unique physiologies. Personally, I have scoliosis with 3 S-curvatures at different points on my spine, and rotation of the spine as well. This means I have a manageable amount of chronic aching, and that there are some moves that feel better to me than others (for instance, heavy deadlifts or back squats do not feel comfortable because one of my curvatures is near the hip, where we hinge for those movements). Other times, I have a flare up of a skeletal/muscular/tendon issue that I got from my first pregnancy. I am vigilant in doing stretching and mobility exercises that I have learned help with my area, but I still need to modify certain movements, and that's okay. In fact, it's smart, because we are in this game for longevity, and if we injure ourselves, we take ourselves out of the game.

Time & Mood

Some of us are morning larks, others are night owls. Sometimes we have the ability to work out when we are feeling our freshest and most energetic, but other times we don't. Depending on how we feel at the time of day when we are working out, we may need to modify our movements or intensity level.

Our emotions also play a role. I don't know about you, but exercise is a definite stress reliever for me. Even when I don't "want" to, regardless of whether my stress is from a hard day at work, family dynamics, or conflict, exercise *always* makes me feel better. Sometimes that means I want a long walk alone, or pushing heavy weight, or even a methodical plodding through several movements. Do what feels good in the moment. Use the workout levels as starting points for you to mix and match what peaks your interest that day.

Equipment & Location

I have used these workouts when I'm at home – and therefore have access to some equipment – but I've also used them while traveling, which could mean no equipment at all, or whatever the hotel gym has on hand. Use the levels to pick and choose what works for wherever you are.

The bottom line is, look through the workout levels, then mix and match to your heart's content.

5

SETTING UP

A lright! Now that we've set the groundwork as to the importance of these workouts and how to maximize them, let's get you ready to use them!

Tracking

The high intensity workouts in this book use minimal equipment, and every workout will offer some variation of movements that won't require any at all (the "Keep Me Moving" levels will always be equipment free; see Chapter 8). You will be able to find modifications and complete the workouts no matter where you are! Use the levels to help modify the workouts to suit your needs & situation each day.

One idea to consider, if you enjoy tracking progress like I do, is to put a checkmark next to the workouts you do (and/or the date), as well as any modifications you make.

Of course, you can use your own journal / fitness log if you keep one. You can do the workouts in order (like I will), and you have the flexibility to move things around. Feel free to repeat a few, mix and match, or try them all!

Timer

The workouts will often require a timer. I like to use the SmartWod timer on my phone. Check out the app store for others. You'll need one that can handle AMRAP, For Time, Tabata, and EMOM / Intervals.

Equipment & Space

Many options require none. Other equipment is minimal. Here is a list of equipment I have used doing these workouts:

- Resistance bands

- Dumbbells (or you can get creative with jugs of rice/water),

- Bench / solid chair

- Box

- Jump rope

- Pull up bar over door / table

- Kettlebell

- Yoga mat / towel for the floor

The majority of these workouts require no more than a small space inside your garage or home. A small square is usually more than enough – you'll need enough space for you to not touch anything with your arms and legs outstretched.

The only other space you might need is a sidewalk / road for walking and running. If you have a cardio machine at home, like a treadmill, stationary bike, or erg, feel free to use that when the workout calls for running (it's often listed for you as an option already).

6

KEY TERMS & DEFINITIONS

In order to familiarize yourself with the lingo used in these workouts, here is a quick glossary of terms for you. Feel free to refer back to this when you can't quite recall what something means.

WORKOUTS

Each workout has a "style" or flow. Below are the terms you'll find in these workouts, their explanations, and an example from the workouts provided.

EMOM (Every Minute on the Minute) — This means that at the top of every minute, you will complete the work (movements) provided. The number following shows how many minutes you will do the movement(s). You could be doing several movements each minute, or just one each minute and rotate through. Once you finish the movement for that minute, you rest the remaining time of that 60 second window.

Examples

EMOM 10

- 2 push ups

- 4 sit ups

- 6 air squats

Every minute for 10 minutes, you perform 2 push ups, 4 sit ups, and 6 air squats. If that takes you 40 seconds, you rest for 20 seconds before the second minute begins.

Note: This workout is not in the charts, so consider this a bonus for you! It's short but gets intense.

EMOM 12

- Min 1: 8 alternating V-ups

- Min 2: 10 burpees

- Min 3: 12 jumping squats

The first minute, you perform 8 alternating V ups and rest until minute 2 begins. The second minute, you do 10 burpees and rest the remaining time. Minute three, you do 12 jumping squats and rest. When minute 4 begins, you repeat from the top. In this workout, you would perform each movement four times.

Ascending / Descending Ladders — These workouts move up or down a "ladder", where you perform one more (or less) repetition than the last time.

Ladders could start with 1 rep and move up (ascending), or start with the higher rep count and move down (descending), or do both. Reps can jump by 1-2 reps each time.

Example:

Descending & Ascending Ladder

10-9-8-7-6-5-4-3-2-1

- Up downs

- Crunches

400m jog or rest 2 minutes

1-2-3-4-5-6-7-8-9-10

- Up downs

- Crunches

This workout has you doing 10 up downs, then 10 crunches, followed by 9 reps of up downs, then 9 of crunches, then 8 and 8, decreasing by one each round, until you complete one of each movement. You complete the 400m run as an active break, and then begin to go back up the ladder: 1 up down and 1 crunch, 2 up downs and 2 crunches, 3 and 3, etc, until you get to 10.

AMRAP (As Many Rounds / Reps as Possible) — This workout flow means you are trying to complete as many rounds or reps of the movements as you can in the time indicated. Once you complete all the reps of each movement, you begin again from the top as long as there is still time remaining. Rest as needed.

Example:

AMRAP 15

- 5 bent over rows

- 10 knee push-ups

- 30 alternating lunges, 15 each leg

This workout will have you moving for 15 minutes, doing 5 bent over rows, 10 knee push ups, and 30 alternating lunges as one round. Once you finish a round, you start again with 5 bent over rows and keep moving through all reps and movements, resting as needed, for 15 minutes.

Intervals — Intervals can vary in time, but it simply means that you are moving for a certain time period, and resting for a time period.

Example:

Intervals :45 sec on, :15 sec off x5 rounds

- Knee push ups

- Tricep dips on a chair

- Sumo air squats

- Plank hold

- Russian twists

You are completing each movement for 45 seconds, then transitioning/resting to the next movement during the 15 second rest period. Complete five rounds total of all five movements. The workout would be 25 minutes total.

21-15-9 — Similar to a descending ladder, you perform 21 repetitions of all movements, then 15 of all movements, and then 9 of each movement. You perform one at a time, so that instead of doing 45 reps all at once, you break them up in three descending rounds.

Example:

21-15-9

- Romanian DL

- Reverse lunges x2

- Bent over row (alternate as needed)

- Push press

This means you complete 21 reps of Romanian deadlifts, 21 reverse lunges each leg (x2 means one each leg, so 42 total), 21 bent over rows, switching arms as needed, and 21 push press. Then you go to 15 reps of each movement, then finish with 9 reps of each movement.

TABATA — Tabata is 8 rounds of :20 seconds of work, and :10 seconds of rest, for 4 minutes total. Typically, you focus on one movement for all 8 rounds, but you can alternate two moves for four rounds each. It doesn't sound like a lot of work, but it is! Give it your all for those 20 seconds of work.

Example:

TABATA x4

- Push ups

- Mountain climbers

- Sit Ups

- Skater slides

Rest one minute between each movement

Complete 8 :20 rounds of push ups, rest one minute. Complete eight :20 rounds of mountain climbers. Rest one minute. Complete eight :20 rounds of sit ups. Rest one minute. Complete eight :20 rounds of skater slides. Done.

ROUNDS FOR TIME — Instead of working out for a specific number of minutes, you complete the specified number of rounds, regardless of time it takes to finish. You complete the repetitions of each movement in each round, then continue repeating those reps and movements until you have finished the designated number of rounds. Rest as needed.

Example:

FIVE ROUNDS FOR TIME

- 40 penguin hops

- 30 suitcase lunges

- 20 sit ups

- 10 DB thrusters

Here you would start with 40 penguin hops, move to 30 suitcase lunges, 20 sit ups, and 10 dumbbell thrusters to complete one round. Repeat the 40-30-20-10 for the second round, and continue until five rounds are complete.

MOVEMENTS

These are the movements you will see in the warm up and workouts, listed in alphabetical order. To see demonstrations, visit the link provided or google the movement.

- 1 0 0 s : https://youtu.be/_ddZRBGG6p0?si=sJfho9or-LYZBtbzK

Begin by lying on the mat. Bend your knees into your chest and lift your head and shoulders off the Mat. Extend your legs out to a high diagonal and reach your arms long by your side with palms facing down. Arms *pump* vigorously, lifting up and down no higher than the hips. Be sure your lower back pushes into the ground and doesn't arch off the mat. You may keep the legs bent in a table top position. To increase difficulty, extend the legs in a high diagonal or lower them keeping them as close to the mat as possible without touching it.

- A - s k i p s : https://youtu.be/O9wh-huxbxU?si=2ENO_IriBFDv5p2t Start position: Stand with your feet hip-width apart, look straight ahead, and keep your upper body tall. Drive right knee up to hip height while pushing up on the ball of your left foot, coming up onto the toe. Land your foot slightly below your hips, and shift weight so that you can drive your left knee up as high as it can go, pushing up onto the right toe. Repeat. Can be done moving forward or stationary. (Arms are bent, elbows tucked in and follow leg movements.)

- **Bench / Chest press:** https://youtu.be/1V3vp-caxRYQ?si=JVMCEtdIiMCItJGk While lying on a bench, extend the weights over your chest with straight arms. Lower both dumbbells to the chest before extending the arms to press them back up again.

- ○ Floor press: Lie on the ground if you don't have a bench. Shorter range of motion but still works the area!

- **Bent   over   row:** https://youtu.be/VP_f9V854og?si=_PWvGM8j7lrDo38Z Begin with your legs shoulder width apart, knees slightly bent. With a dumbbell in each hand, palms facing each other, bend over at a 45-degree angle and inhale. Pull the dumbbells up towards the outside of your chest / ribs as you exhale. Lift to the point your range of motion allows. Slowly lower weights as you inhale. Stay bent over until reps are complete, keeping your spine neutral and tailbone pointing toward the wall behind you.

- **Box   Jumps:** https://youtu.be/NBY9-kTuHEk?si=Zd55Qs-rNSj9P2El Facing the box, place your feet about 6 inches from the box, hip-width apart. Bend your knees and send your hips back as you swing your arms behind you ,then explosively push through the balls of your feet, jumping straight up, swinging your arms forward to get as much height as possible. To land, bend your knees again and land with both feet on top. Stand straight up on top of the box, then step down for the next rep. If using a bench or chair, make sure it is sturdy and won't move as you're trying to land on it.

- **Bicycle crunch:** https://www.verywellfit.com/bicycle-crunch-exercise-3120058 Lie flat on the floor with lower back pressed to the ground and knees bent. Contract your abdomen to stabilize your spine. Place hands behind head, pull shoulders back, and raise knees to a 90-degree angle off the floor. As you exhale, bring one knee towards your armpit while straightening your other leg, keeping both knees higher than your hips. Rotate your torso to touch your elbow to the opposite knee as it comes up. Repeat while twisting to the other side.

- **Boot Strappers**: https://youtu.be/-SAna4vOJhA?si=14VCZ8vtgyWuHb6q Start in a squat position with your hands grabbing the toes of your feet. Straighten your legs to lift your hips into the air, stretching your hamstrings, while keeping your hands on your feet. Then, lower back into the squat position and repeat the movement. Feel free to hold the top or bottom of the stretch, shift weight from foot to foot, or other small moves that feel good to your body.

- **Burpees:** https://youtu.be/auBLPXO8Fww?si=BizOHloUmlhYclFUFrom a standing position, place feet shoulder-width apart. Squat down, placing your hands on the ground in front of you. From there, kick your legs back to get into a push-up (plank) position. Lower your entire body to the ground so your chest and thighs are touching the ground. Next, jump or step your feet forward toward your hands, returning to the squat position. Finally, slightly jump up into the air with your hands raised above your head.

- ○ **Push Up Burpee:** Be strict in your movement - from the plank position, keep your body straight as you do a push-up by lowering your chest to the ground, then pushing back up into plank position before standing back up for the jump.

- **Crunches:** https://youtu.be/RUNrHkbP4Pc?si =JgaNoCjGSRzEE7FjLie flat on your back with your knees bent and feet flat on the floor. Place your hands behind your head, without pulling on your neck. Engage your core muscles, and lift your upper body off the floor, bringing your shoulders toward your knees. Keep your lower back on the ground and avoid using momentum. Once your upper body is lifted a few inches, pause briefly, then slowly lower yourself back down to the starting position.

- **Deadlift (w/ Dumbbell):** https://youtu.be/JN-pUNRPQkAk?si=Jm0SHo3pNaiA6iFS Start by standing with your feet shoulder-width apart, holding a dumbbell in each hand with your arms at your sides. Keep your back straight and your chest up as you hinge at the hips, pushing your hips back while bending your knees into almost a half squat. Lower the dumbbells toward the ground, keeping them close to your body, until you feel a stretch in your hamstrings. Make sure to keep your head in a neutral position, looking slightly ahead. Then, push through your heels and engage your glutes to stand back up, bringing the dumbbells back to the starting position.

- ○ **Romanian Deadlift:** https://youtu.be/UsO jCcxSJaI?si=zTet6UxCMfh640lTKnees have a very slight bend and back is straight as you hinge at the hips, not the knees. Push your hips back while lowering the dumbbells along the *front* of your legs. Focus on keeping the weights close to your body, lowering them until you feel a stretch in your hamstrings, usually around mid-shins. Keep chest up and shoulders back throughout the movement. To return to the starting position, push through your heels and engage your glutes to stand up straight, bringing the dumbbells back to your sides.

- **Devils Press:** https://youtu.be/zlqEtAUds-I?si= VwcWqJmlxrB3wilEPlace a pair of dumbbells on the floor in front of you, around shoulder-width apart, and stand with your feet shoulder-width apart. Bend at your hips and knees to lower your body, placing hands on the dumbbells. Kick your feet back to get into a push-up position. Perform a push-up by lowering your chest to the ground, then push back up to the starting plank position. Immediately after the push-up, jump your feet forward to your hands, returning to a squat position with the dumbbells still in hand. From the squat, explosively stand up and press the dumbbells overhead in one fluid motion. Lower the dumbbells back to the starting position.

- **Double Unders:** https://youtu.be/-tF3hUsPZAI?si=T9DMZzNSJZV3ff5kBegin by performing a standard jump to get into a rhythm. As you jump, use your wrists to rotate the rope quickly, aiming to make two rotations of the rope for every jump. Jump slightly higher than you would for a single under to allow the rope to pass under your feet twice. Focus on keeping your elbows close to your sides and using your wrists for the rope's motion rather than your arms. Land softly on the balls of your feet to maintain balance and prepare for the next jump.

- **Glute bridge:** https://youtu.be/tqp5XQPp-TxY?si=VmtXwMgUoVyYgiNS To do a glute bridge, lie on your back with your knees bent, feet flat on the floor, and arms by your sides. Push through your heels and lift your hips off the ground, squeezing your glutes at the top, forming a straight line from your shoulders to your knees. Hold briefly, then lower your hips back down with control, and repeat.

- **Goblet march:** https://youtu.be/aAFF0WrHnfU?si=Q-kP_hiJDrRO8yZCHold a dumbbell or kettlebell close to (but not touching) your chest in a "goblet" grip. Stand tall with your feet hip-width apart, engage your core, and lift one knee toward your chest while maintaining balance. Lower your leg, then lift the other knee in a marching motion. Continue alternating legs, or walk forward, keeping your posture straight and the weight secure by your chest. You may rest the weight on your chest to make it easier.

- **Good Mornings:** https://youtu.be/nczH_7m1TnI?si=OUdsWECDC7j2vFOiStand with your feet hip-width apart with hands behind your head. Keep your back straight and knees slightly bent as you hinge at your hips. Keep your core engaged as you lower your torso until it's almost parallel to the ground. Engage your glutes and hamstrings to lift your torso back to the starting position.

- **High   Pull:** https://youtu.be/oOKJD3Xn3fc?si=DOwHDnD-horWqfBKu When the dumbbells are in front of your thighs, pull them up toward your chin while keeping your elbows higher than your wrists. At the top of the movement, your elbows should be pointing outward and upward while the dumbbells are close to your chest. Lower the weights in a controlled manner.

- **Hollow Hold:** https://youtu.be/p7j02V1fIzU?si=g0cE0sFWcD3cizewLie on your back with your arms extended overhead and legs straight. Engage your core, lift your shoulders and legs off the ground, creating a curved "hollow" shape with your body. Keep your lower back pressed into the floor and hold this position while maintaining tension in your abs.

- **Inchworms:** https://youtu.be/ZY2ji_Ho0dA?si=Au_FNXkaa2uzdnN4Start by standing tall, then bend at your hips to place your hands on the floor in front of you, keeping legs straight. Walk your hands forward into a plank position, keeping your legs as straight as possible. After reaching a plank, walk your feet toward your hands, returning to a standing position. Repeat the movement, alternating between walking your hands and feet forward. Alternately, you can do a "stationary" version by walking your hands out as far as they can go, then walking your hands back in, all while keeping legs as straight as possible.

- **Jumping jacks:** https://youtu.be/2W4ZNSwoW_4?si=QH5RBndmptN1ZPVAStanding with your feet together and arms by your sides, jump while spreading your legs out to the sides and raising your arms overhead. Jump again to bring your feet back together and lower your arms to your sides. Repeat the movement continuously, keeping a steady rhythm.

- **Kettlebell swing:** https://youtu.be/mKDIuUbH94Q?si=h32hz_GR8U5lnenrTo do a kettlebell swing, stand with your feet shoulder-width apart, holding the kettlebell with both hands in front of you. Hinge at your hips, keeping your back straight, and swing the kettlebell slightly behind you between your legs. Drive through your hips and stand up explosively, swinging the kettlebell to chest height (or straight overhead if you are experienced). Let it swing back down between your legs, and repeat, maintaining a strong core and controlled motion.

- **Russian:** https://youtu.be/_vtp1QiJjeY?si=c P7AWswL6lI6I0zb - stays at forehead height, recommended for anyone with a history of shoulder issues.

- **Dumbbell swing:** https://youtu.be/uB-fq 0HqGK0?si=VmpgTRgPT1Akm0H7 - raise only to forehead height, do NOT go overhead with a dumbbell.

- **Lizard Lunge:** https://youtu.be/jXk5dquBT6 w?si=NmBY1rc-iCvC_QPxBegin in a plank position, then step your right foot outside your right hand, lowering your hips toward the floor. Keep your back leg extended and your core engaged as you feel the stretch in your hips and thighs. Hold the position, then switch sides by stepping your left foot outside your left hand to stretch the other side.

- **Lunge Stretch with Thoracic Rotation:** https://youtu.be/BxLkf1V0M94?si=Kw0L 4azgqWUDhCduSame instructions as lizard lunge. When right foot is forward and right hand is planted inside the right foot, rotate your left hand and arm straight up to the ceiling. When you switch to the left foot forward and left hand planted inside the left foot, rotate the right hand straight up to the ceiling to get the twist in the spine.

- **Lunges (Walking):** https://youtu.be/L8fvypPrz zs?si=MgF6AhnzKQdaBT7dStart by standing tall with your feet hip-width apart. Step forward with one leg, lowering your hips until both knees are bent at 90-degree angles. Keep your front knee aligned with your ankle and your back knee just above the floor. Push through your front heel to return to the starting position, then switch legs and repeat, or walk forward as you lunge.

  - **Jumping:** https://youtu.be/I4mIS7p6EfU?si =L6AhFyPcqF0bvFya - stay stationary but explode as you come upwards so that your feet leave the ground slightly.

  - **Suitcase:** https://youtu.be/KOLD4DlhJ64?s i=9vTdAEflar6z_-dh - holding one or two dumbbells straight down to your side as you lunge.

  - **Reverse:** https://youtu.be/xrPteyQLGAo?si =BNcNOY3r5f__JuEn - stepping backward instead of forward

- **Mountain climbers:** https://youtu.be/zT-9L 3CEcmk?si=XWFQANfTnIMk05G0Start in a plank position with your hands directly under your shoulders. Quickly drive one knee toward your chest, then switch legs, bringing the other knee forward while pushing the first leg back. Continue alternating knees at a quick pace, keeping your core engaged and maintaining a straight line from your head to your heels.

- **Penguin hops:** https://youtu.be/XA5SbAIRNFg?si=NEoTyGJw-dBDGzUWBegin by standing with your feet shoulder-width apart. Jump off the ground keeping a slight bend in your legs, and, as you jump, tap your thighs with both hands twice before landing. Focus on keeping your jumps low and quick while maintaining a steady rhythm. Repeat the movement, aiming to perform the taps efficiently with each jump.

- **Plank:** https://youtu.be/J3QKdw79lNw?si=I8bSVVjq7yBFyXXCStart by getting into a push-up position with your forearms on the ground and your body in a straight line from head to heels. Engage your core, keep your back flat, and hold this position without letting your hips drop. You can also straighten your arms into a high plank, making sure your hands are directly under your shoulders.

  - **Diagonal plank:** https://youtu.be/OGfFtF-dhrk?si=Jyr2ERSu0MhTsQ2VStarting from plank position, widen the feet slightly. Lift the left arm and right leg into the air simultaneously while maintaining neutral hip position, keeping their movement to a minimum.

Hold them in the air briefly, then lower them slowly, with control, to the starting position. Alternate.

- **Pull throughs:** https://youtu.be/Zko5x2SoQmo?si=n-KQHJUUrMYCMc9aIn a plank position with a dumbbell placed outside your right arm, reach with the left hand underneath the body to grab the dumbbell, pulling it across the floor to the opposite side of your body, all while keeping your hips stable and avoiding any twisting. Alternate sides, pulling the dumbbell through with the other hand, while maintaining a strong plank position and minimizing hip rotation.

- **Side plank:** https://youtu.be/2W96p2PIoPg?si=UsdaD4j2QhhGT8XULie on your side with your legs stacked and your elbow directly under your shoulder. Lift your hips off the ground, forming a straight line from your head to your feet. Engage your core and hold this position, ensuring your body stays aligned and stable. Switch sides when ready.

- **Kneeling Side Plank with Leg Lift:** https://youtu.be/MdjSIC7SgoE?si=Z3fEZ8eUW-sZ819EBegin by kneeling on one knee with your other leg extended straight out to the side and your foot flat on the floor. Place your elbow directly under your shoulder and lift your hips off the ground into a side plank position. From here, raise your extended leg upwards while keeping your body stable, engaging your core and glutes. Lower your leg back down with control and repeat for the desired number of repetitions before switching sides.

- ○ **Walks (Lateral):** https://youtu.be/yCVya X-RjLM?si=FdxqLLeUStVPYCGStart in a plank position with your hands directly under your shoulders and your body in a straight line. Keeping your core engaged, step your right hand and right foot out to the side, then follow with your left hand and left foot to return to a wide plank position. Repeat the movement by stepping back to the center and alternating sides, maintaining a strong plank posture throughout.

- **Pull ups:** https://youtu.be/HRV5YKKaeVw?si= haJkt8H9qyxOD2spStart by gripping a pull-up bar with your hands slightly wider than shoulder-width apart and your palms facing away from you (overhand grip). Hang from the bar with your arms fully extended and your feet off the ground. Engage your core and pull your shoulder blades down and back to stabilize your body. Then, bend your elbows and pull your chin above the bar, focusing on using your back and arm muscles. Keep your body straight and avoid swinging or using momentum. Once your chin is over the bar, lower yourself back down with control until your arms are fully extended again.

○ **Table pull ups:** https://youtu.be/woGSKA2tPrY?si=VNhsDEdfGkI9zTsuStart by lying on your back underneath a sturdy table or a low bar, with your head facing the table's underside. Reach up and grip the edge of the table with both hands, positioning your hands shoulder-width apart. Keep your body straight and your feet flat on the ground or elevated on another surface (elevated feet will be more challenging). Engage your core and pull your chest toward the table, bending your elbows and squeezing your shoulder blades together. Use your arms and back muscles to lift your body while maintaining a straight line from your head to your heels. Once your chest touches or comes close to the table, lower yourself back down with control until your arms are fully extended.

• **Push press:** https://youtu.be/4tCaD42ghlc?si=suMTSGtil8HXfum9Stand with feet shoulder-width apart, holding a dumbbell in each hand at shoulder height, with your palms facing forward. Begin by slightly bending your knees and engaging your core for stability. Then, push through your legs as you explosively extend your knees and hips, using that momentum to press the dumbbells overhead. Keep your elbows close to your body as you lift, and ensure that your arms are fully extended at the top of the movement. Hold the position briefly, then lower the dumbbells back to shoulder height in a controlled manner.

- **Push ups:** https://youtu.be/0pkjOk0EiAk?si=1GsBJ2VFoUYNtwXuOn the floor, place your hands *slightly* wider than shoulder-width apart, with your fingers pointing forward. Push yourself up onto your toes, keeping your body in a straight line from head to heels. Engage your core and lower your body toward the ground by bending your elbows, keeping elbows close to your sides. Lower yourself until your chest touches the floor, then push through your hands to raise your body back to the starting position. Make sure to keep your back straight throughout the movement.

    - **Chair push ups:** https://youtu.be/kJ5CpP_Vjdo?si=F-FXKx5zgsn7CBSRDone while putting hands on the edge a sturdy chair

    - **Knee push ups:** https://youtu.be/jWxvty2KROs?si=GOsFZGyg4zEtrtQ0Same form, but put knees on ground

    - **Pike push ups:** https://youtu.be/XckEEwa1BPI?si=ZJ-mFAD0xzBN9ctFStart in a downward dog position with your hands placed shoulder-width apart on the floor and your feet hip-width apart. Lift your hips up and back, forming an upside-down "V" shape with your body. From this position, bend your elbows and lower your head toward the ground, aiming to touch the floor between your hands. Keep your legs straight and your core engaged as you lower and lift your body. Once the top of your head is near or at the ground, push back up to return to the starting position.

- ○ **Wall push ups:** https://youtu.be/-KVhap nEtuk?si=ALHzqcMUidN4QbWiDone while putting hands on a wall

- **Russian twist:** https://youtu.be/JyUqwkVpsi8?si=6ZDrkoD5yfmf0L17Sit on the floor with your knees bent and your feet flat. Lean back slightly while keeping your back straight, engaging your core. You can hold your hands together in front of you or grasp a weight for added resistance. Lift your feet off the ground so that shins are parallel to the floor, balancing on your sit bones. Rotate your torso to the right, bringing your hands or the weight beside your hip, then twist back to the center and rotate to the left. Continue alternating sides in a controlled manner, focusing on engaging your abdominal muscles

- **Shoulder taps:** https://youtu.be/C6At19Q9i2Q?si=YQG0wIJTALj_4WDXStart in a plank position with your hands directly under your shoulders and your body in a straight line from head to heels. Engage your core to keep your hips stable as you lift one hand off the ground and tap the opposite shoulder. Make sure to keep your body as still as possible and avoid rotating your hips. Lower your hand back to the floor and repeat the movement with the other hand, tapping the opposite shoulder. Continue alternating sides while maintaining a strong plank position, focusing on controlling your movements and keeping your core tight throughout the exercise.

- **Sit up:** https://youtu.be/Q15ClFuxfeM?si=ZO4 qyLnzII6hVft_Start by lying flat on your back with your knees bent and feet flat on the floor, about hip-width apart. Cross your arms over your chest or place your hands behind your head, making sure not to pull on your neck. Engage your core and use your abdominal muscles to lift your upper body off the ground, rolling up toward your knees. Aim to sit all the way up until your torso is vertical and shoulders are aligned with or past your hips. Hold the position briefly at the top, then slowly lower your upper body back down to the starting position with control.

- **Skater slides:** https://youtu.be/Jx2KXGbQkY M?si=_nYZBhoyhND4rA8UStand with your feet shoulder-width apart, bend your knees slightly and shift your weight onto your right leg. From this position, push off with your right foot and jump to the left, landing on your left foot while bringing your right foot behind your left leg, similar to a skating motion. As you land, bend your left knee to absorb the impact and keep your core engaged for stability. Immediately push off from your left foot to jump to the right, landing on your right foot and bringing your left foot behind your right leg. You can keep the back foot raised or tap it to the ground if you need stability or balance. Continue alternating sides in a smooth, controlled motion, focusing on maintaining balance and proper form throughout the exercise.

- **Snatch:** https://youtu.be/9520DJiFmvE?si=7Qu qHPPyIrajMrPvStart by standing with your feet shoulder-width apart, holding a dumbbell in one hand on the floor between your feet. Bend your knees and hinge at your hips to lower your body while keeping your back straight. Grab the dumbbell with one hand, then explosively extend your hips and legs, driving the dumbbell upward. As the dumbbell rises, pull it close to your body and rotate your wrist to bring it overhead in one fluid motion. Finish by locking your arm out overhead, with your body in a straight line from your heels to your hands. Lower the dumbbell back down to the starting position and repeat, or switch to the other hand if alternating. Make sure to maintain control throughout the movement and keep your core engaged for stability.

- **Squats (air):** https://youtu.be/kTdNI6Alh4c? si=OrU2GVNdL2xIVJ3eStand with your feet shoulder-width apart and your toes slightly pointed out. Keep your chest up and your core engaged as you bend your knees and push your hips back, like you're sitting down into a chair. Lower yourself until your thighs are parallel to the floor or slightly below, making sure your knees stay aligned with your toes. Press through your heels to stand back up, fully extending your legs to return to the starting position. Maintain good posture and control throughout.

- **Banded** - put a resistance band around your legs, above your knees

- **Chair** - squat to a chair behind you

- **Goblet** - hold a dumbbell or kettlebell in your hands at chest level as you squat

- **Jumping squat** - keep the same squat technique, but explode up as you rise so that your feet come up off the floor

- **Sumo squat:** https://youtu.be/vBA3vyOxJv0?si=QAFvU_QOvfdoyiHd - move your feed into a wider position (outside the shoulders) as you squat

- **Starburst jumps:** STAR BURST To do a starburst jump, start by standing with your feet together and your arms at your sides. Lower into as low of a squat as possible with arms tucked by your feed, then jump explosively into the air. While jumping, spread your arms and legs out wide, creating a star shape with your body. As you land softly, bring your feet back together and your arms to your sides, returning to the starting position. Repeat the movement, focusing on making a controlled, wide "burst" each time you jump.

- **Step ups:** https://youtu.be/5qjqDHOUh-A?si=1 tBYEdL3z309xE—Start by standing in front of a sturdy bench or step, with your feet hip-width apart. Place your right foot firmly on the step, making sure your entire foot is on the surface. Engage your core and push through your right heel to lift your body up, bringing your left foot up to the step until you're standing tall. Make sure to keep your back straight and your chest up throughout the movement. To return to the starting position, step back down with your left foot, followed by your right foot, returning to the ground. Alternate by repeating with the other foot first.

- **Strict Press (Dumbbell Press):** https://youtu.be/AqzDJHxyn-wo?si=kpM6wkwYFJQD7VLr Stand with your feet hip-width apart and hold a dumbbell in each hand at shoulder height, with your palms facing forward and elbows bent. Keeping your core tight, chest lifted, and back straight, and without using momentum or bending your knees, press the dumbbells directly overhead until your arms are fully extended. Keep your wrists in line with your shoulders. Slowly lower the dumbbells back to the starting position in a controlled manner.

  ○ Seated Press: The exact same move, but seated on the ground or a bench. This removes all lower body momentum and forces only the upper body to do the work. You will likely need a lighter weight.

- **S u p e r m e n :** https://youtu.be/z6PJMT2y8GQ?si=7Gzl-hoZGILPGmh_z To do a Superman hold, lie face down on the floor with your arms extended straight out in front of you and your legs fully stretched out. Engage your core and lower back muscles as you lift your arms, chest, and legs off the ground at the same time, holding them up as high as you can while also lengthening. Engage the core. Keep your neck neutral and look slightly ahead, not straight up. Hold this position, feeling the tension in your back and glutes, then slowly lower your arms and legs back to the floor.

- **Toe   taps:** https://youtu.be/Ml2xTP45jVQ?si=4MRrBOBf-pgDN4RO9 Lie flat on your back with your legs bent in a table top position, knees at 90 degrees. Place your hands beneath your low back, behind the head, or straight out on either side of you. Be sure you are pressing your low back into the ground. Engage your core and lift your shoulders and upper back off the ground, lower one leg toward the ground and tap the toe to the floor before returning to table top. Alternate legs while keeping shoulders off the ground.

  - **Extended   Leg:**

https://www.painscale.com/article/core-strength-leg-extension Straighten each leg as you lower, instead of keeping the knee bent.

- **Tricep dips:** https://youtu.be/0326dy_-CzM?si=e_7Z9tHl2-BAhtns Sit on the edge of a stable chair or bench and grip the edge of it outside your hips with your hands. Fingers pointed at feet, legs extended, and feet a few inches apart, heels touching ground. Look straight ahead, keeping chin up. Press into your palms to lift your body and slide forward far enough that your bum is past the edge of the chair. Slowly lower yourself down until your elbows are bent to a 90 degree angle. Push yourself back up until your arms are straight, and repeat. Can bend knees for a slightly easier variation.

- **Thrusters:** https://youtu.be/u3wKkZjE8QM?si=1_k8yhYiH2FhefGpStart by standing with your feet shoulder-width apart, holding a pair of dumbbells with palms facing inward. Squat down, keeping your chest up and pushing your hips back until your thighs are parallel to the floor. From the squat, drive through your heels to stand up explosively while pressing the weights overhead in one smooth motion. As you straighten your legs, fully extend your arms above your head. Lower the weights back to your shoulders and immediately go into the next squat for the next repetition.

- **Up downs:** https://youtu.be/4NRFUKgNhs8?si =K_SL8P_o2xXR0GooA warm up or modification for burpees. Start by standing with your feet shoulder-width apart. Quickly drop into a squat position and place your hands on the ground in front of you. From there, kick your legs straight back to get into a plank position, keeping your body straight. Immediately jump your feet back towards your hands, returning to the squat position. Then, stand back up without the jump, completing one repetition.

- **V-ups:** https://youtu.be/7UVgs18Y1P4?si=8Fgb7 TTA6OC9qZ80 To do a V-up, lie flat on your back with your legs straight and arms extended overhead. Engage your core and lift your legs and upper body off the ground at the same time, reaching your hands toward your toes. Your body will form a "V" shape as you balance on your hips. Try to keep your legs straight and reach as high as you can. After touching your toes or getting as close as possible, lower your arms and legs back down in a controlled motion without letting them touch the ground, and then repeat the movement.

  - **Alternating:** Lift only one leg a time while maintaining the other one straight on the ground.

7

THE WORKOUTS

Before you start working out, it's important to warm up your body. There are different perspectives on this, but I think stretching is best done AFTER a workout. Using movement to warm up your body is the best way to get ready for these workouts. You can do an easy warm up, find your own, or follow those provided.

WARM UPS

No Thinking Warm Up:

Walk, bike, row or jog for 3-5 minutes to warm up.

Focused Warmup:

Perform 1-2 rounds of this before every workout:

- 30 lateral hops (side to side on the floor, or over a dumbbell)

- 10 good mornings

- 10 bootstrappers

- 30 second hold at bottom of last bootstrapper, lengthening spine and pushing hips down or knees out with elbows

- 5 inchworms with push-up and down dog stretch

- 5 lizard lunge stretch each leg (option to add thoracic rotation)

- 5 light dumbbell deadlifts each arm

- 5 light dumbbell shoulder press each arm

- 10 air squats / goblet squats (light weight)

LEVELED CHARTS EXPLANATION

Ideally, the more intense workouts in this book are partnered with monostructural / cardiovascular exercises, like swimming, running, or biking, throughout the week. The chart below offers suggestions for what those might look like, as well as time duration, for each level. As always, you use your own discretion as to what will work for you. You know yourself best.

Cardiovascular Conditioning Workouts (2-3x a week)	Keep Me Moving	Kick It Up A Notch	Turbo Boost Me
Brisk walking (like you're late) Bicycling / Rowing Hiking Dancing Hot Yoga / Pilates	10-15 minutes	20-30 minutes	45+ minutes
Swimming (freestyle, backstroke, breaststroke, butterfly)	5-10 minutes	15-20 minutes	25+ minutes

WORKOUTS

Now we've come to the list of workouts! Each chart is organized by week, with three high intensity workouts each week. You'll see the workout format in the first column, and then three options on the right to complete them: *Keep Me Moving, Kick It Up a Notch*, and *Turbo Boost Me*. If you read across from left to right, you'll notice that each movement has "progressions" to take it heavier or more intense at the next level. Read through each level, then choose your workout according to your current needs and options (physical space, body, mind, equipment, location).

Remember, you are in control! You pick the order, the level, the movement and use these charts as your guide. The workout descriptions and demonstration links in Chapter 6 whenever you need them. Workout charts begin on the next page. Get to it and have fun!

WEEK ONE			
High Intensity Workouts (2-3x a week)	**Keep Me Moving**	**Kick It Up A Notch**	**Turbo Boost Me**
1 **EMOM 20** Minute 1: first movement Minute 2: second movement Minute 3: third movement Minute 4: fourth movement Minute 5: rest	1. Marching in place 2. Superman holds / pulses 3. Glute bridges 4. Table Pull ups 5. Rest	1. A-skips 2. Superman holds 3. Glute bridges 4. Bent over rows 5. Rest	1. Goblet March 2. Thrusters with DB 3. Glute bridges w/ DB over hips 4. Pull Ups 5. Rest
2 **Descending & Ascending Ladder** 10-9-8-7-6-5-4-3-2-1 Run / row / bike 1-2-3-4-5-6-7-8-9-10 *use cardio portion as active rest or rest if needed	• Up Downs • Toe Taps • 200m run / 300m row / 400m bike (~1 min)	• Burpees • Toe Tap leg extensions • 300m run / 400m row / 500m bike (~90 seconds)	• Pushup Burpees • V-Ups • 400m run / 500m row / 600m bike (~2 min)
3 **AMRAP 15** As many reps as possible in 15 minutes. Rest as needed.	• 5 Wall push ups • 10 Air squats • 20 Alt. lunges. 10 each leg	• 5 Knee push ups • 10 Banded air squats • 30 Alt. lunges, 15 each leg	• 5 Push ups • 10 Goblet squats • 30 Weighted alt. lunges, 15 each leg

WEEK TWO			
High Intensity Workouts	**Keep Me Moving**	**Kick It Up A Notch**	**Turbo Boost Me**
4 **21-15-9** *Optional:* add a 200m jog/bike/row after finishing each number (all 21s, all 15s, and all 9s)	• Good mornings • Chair Squat, then stand & raise arms overhead • Table pull ups • Floor press	• Romanian Deadlift • Squat, then stand with toe raise, stretch arms overhead • Bent over row • Bench press	• Romanian Deadlift • Thrusters with DB • Pull Ups • Bench Press
5 **Sprints X10** Choose running, rowing or biking. Stick with the same movement for all 10 rounds, giving max effort.	• 50m run / 100m row / 150m bike • Rest 1 minute • Repeat 9 times	• 75m run / 125m row / 175m bike • Rest 1 minute • Repeat 9 times	• 100m run/ 150m row/ 200m bike • Rest 1 minute • Repeat 9 times
6 **Part One:** 3 Rounds of: Side Planks & Plank holds *Total work time:* 3:00-4:30 **Part Two:** Intervals x5 Rounds :45 sec on, :15 sec off *Total:* 20 minutes	• :20 sec side plank on knees (Left) • :20 side on Right • :20 Plank hold on knees **Part Two:** • Knee push ups • Up Downs • Sumo air squats • Russian twists	• :30 sec side plank on L • :30 side plank on R • :30 Front Plank hold **Part Two:** • Push ups • Russian KBS • Sumo squats • Russian twists	• :30 sec side kneeling side plank w/ leg lift left side • :30 right side • :30 Front Plank hold **Part Two:** • Push ups • Full KBS • Sumo squats w/ high pull • Russian twists (weighted)

WEEK THREE			
High Intensity Workouts	**Keep Me Moving**	**Kick It Up A Notch**	**Turbo Boost Me**
7 **AMRAP 20** As many reps as possible in 20 minutes. Rest as needed.	• 4 Knee push-ups • 8 Walking lunges each leg (16 total) • 12 Bicycle crunches	• 4 Push-ups • 8 Suitcase lunges each leg (1 weight) • 16 Alt toe taps	• 4 Push-ups • 4 Pike push-ups • 16 Walking suitcase lunges (2 weights) • 16 Alt V-ups
8 **EMOM 20-30** Each minute is a different movement. Build in transition to the next movement after 45 or 50 seconds.	**20 MIN** • Jumping Jacks • Tricep dips • Air Squats • Hollow Hold Pulses • Chair Step-ups	**25 MIN** • Penguin Hops • Tricep dips • Banded Squats • Hollow Holds • Box Step Ups	**30 MIN** • Double Unders • Tricep dips • Goblet Squats • Hollow Rocks • Box Jumps
9 **TABATA x4** Do one movement for each Tabata round. Rest one minute between each movement. *Total work time:* 16 minutes	• Starburst Stands • Mountain climbers • Crunches • Table Pull ups	• Starburst Jumps • Mountain climbers • Full Sit ups • Bent Over Row	• Alternating Snatches • Mountain climbers • V-Ups • Pull Ups

WEEK FOUR				
	High Intensity Workouts	**Keep Me Moving**	**Kick It Up A Notch**	**Turbo Boost Me**
10	**4 ROUNDS FOR TIME** Rest as needed.	• 20 Reverse Lunges • 10 Push ups • 10 Good Mornings • 20 Shoulder Taps	• 20 Jumping Lunges • 10 Push up burpees • 10 Romanian Deadlift • 20 Diagonal Planks	• 20 Jumping Lunges • 10 Devils press • 10 Romanian Deadlift • 20 Plank Walks
11	**DOUBLE UP INTERVALS** Do **two** working intervals for each movement before moving on to the next movement. Rest 60 sec after each interval **and** in between each movement at all levels.	*60 seconds of work each interval:* • Skater Steps • 100s: table top position • Air squats *Optional fourth movement: knee plank hold*	*90 seconds of work each interval:* • Skater Slides • 100s: legs extended • Banded Squats *Optional fourth movement: plank hold*	*120 seconds of work each interval:* • Skater Slides • 100s: mix table top and extended • Banded / Goblet Squats • Plank Pull Throughs
12	**Part One:** Five sets, rest 60 sec between sets (Do both moves before rest.) Rest 2-3 minutes, then: **Part Two:** **12 MIN AMRAP**	• 7 pike pushup • 3-5 knee push ups **Part Two:** • 12 Reverse lunges • 10 Step ups • 8 Up downs	• 8 strict press • 4-6 push ups **Part Two:** • 12 Jumping lunges • 10 Box jumps • 8 Burpees	• 7-9 seated press • 5-7 push ups **Part Two:** • 12 Reverse suitcase lunges • 10 Box jumps • 8 Burpees

WEEK FIVE			
High Intensity Workouts	**Keep Me Moving**	**Kick It Up A Notch**	**Turbo Boost Me**
13 **Part One:** 3 Rounds of: Side Planks & Plank holds *Total work time:* 3:00-4:30 **Part Two: AMRAP 18** As many reps as possible in 18 minutes.	• :20 sec side plank on knees (Left) • :20 side on Right • :20 Plank hold on knees **Part Two:** • 4 Push ups • 8 Air Squats + press arms up • 100m run / 200m bike	• :30 sec side plank on L • :30 side plank on R • :30 Front Plank hold **Part Two:** • 6 Push ups • 10 Thrusters • 150m run / 300m bike	• :30 sec side kneeling side plank w/ leg lift left side • :30 right side • :30 Front Plank hold **Part Two:** • 8 Push ups • 12 Thrusters • 200m run / 400m bike
14 **Ascending & Descending Ladder:** 20-18-16-14...2 Rest 2 minutes. 2-4-6-8-10...20	• Good mornings • Crunches • Superman Pulses	• Dumbbell deadlift • Toe Taps • KB / DB Swings	• Dumbbell deadlift • Full sit ups • KB / DB Swings
15 **AMRAP 18/21/24** Rest as needed. **Optional:** Add a 200m run/row or 400m bike after each round.	**18 MIN** • 50 Jumping Jacks • 25 Chair Squats • 10 Up downs • 5 Pike push-ups	**21 MIN** • 75 Single Unders • 25 Air Squats • 10 Burpees • 5 Strict press	**24 MIN** • 50 Double Unders • 25 Banded Squats • 10 Burpees • 5 Seated press

WEEK SIX			
High Intensity Workouts	Keep Me Moving	Kick It Up A Notch	Turbo Boost Me
16 — **ALTERNATING TABATA** Alternate between the two movements for the first round and the other two movements in the second round. **Optional:** *Repeat one or both Tabata Rounds*	First Tabata Round: • Alt Toe Touches • Mountain Climbers Rest 1:00 Second Tabata Round: • Air Squats • Knee push ups	First Tabata Round: • Alternating V-Ups • Mountain Climbers Rest 1:00 Second Tabata Round: • Jumping Squats • Push ups	First Tabata Round: • Double Leg V-Ups • Mountain Climbers Rest 1:00 Second Tabata Round: • Goblet Squats • Pike push ups
17 — Part One: **EMOM 10** Min 1: 1st move Min 2: 2nd move Part Two: 6:00 Intervals x4 rounds: Complete all movements then *rest* the remaining time of the six min. window.	• 8-10 Starbursts • 8-10 Push ups Part Two: • 300m brisk walk / 600m bike • 20 air squats • 30 crunches • 10 pushups	• 10-12 Alt Snatches • 10-12 Floor press Part Two: • 400m jog/row or 600m bike • 20 goblet squats • 20 sit ups • 10 burpees	• 12-14 Alt Snatches • 10-14 Bench press Part Two: • 500m run/row • 20 goblet squats • 30 sit ups • 10 burpees
18 — **FIVE ROUNDS FOR TIME** Rest as needed.	• 40 Jumping Jacks • 30 Lunges • 20 Sit ups • 10 Squats + press arms overhead • 5 Table pull ups	• 40 Penguin Hops • 30 Jumping lunges • 20 Sit ups • 10 DB Thrusters • 5 Bent over row	• 40 Double Unders • 30 Suitcase lunges • 20 Alt V-Ups • 10 DB Thrusters • 5 Pull ups

8

No Equipment Level

"Keep Me Moving" Workouts Only

This chapter provides all the workouts from the "Keep Me Moving" level in one place. No equipment is needed.

1	**EMOM 20** Minute 1: first movement Minute 2: second movement Minute 3: third movement Minute 4: fourth movement Minute 5: rest	• Marching in place • Superman holds / pulses • Glute bridges • Table Pull ups • Rest
2	**Descending & Ascending Ladder** 10-9-8-7-6-5-4-3-2-1 Run / row / bike 1-2-3-4-5-6-7-8-9-10	• Up Downs • Toe Taps • 200m run / 300m row / 400m bike (~1 min) Use cardio portion as active rest or rest instead
3	**AMRAP 15** As many reps as possible in 15 minutes. Rest as needed.	• 5 Wall push ups • 10 Air squats • 20 Alt. lunges, 10 each leg

4	**21-15-9** *Optional:* add a 100m jog/bike/row after finishing each number (all 21s, all 15s, and all 9s)	• Good mornings • Chair Squat, then stand & raise arms overhead • Table pull ups • Floor press
5	**Sprints X10** Choose running, rowing or biking. Stick with the same movement for all 10 rounds, giving max effort.	• 50m run / 100m row / 150m bike • Rest 1 minute • Repeat 9 times
6	**Part One:** 3 Rounds of: Side Planks & Plank holds **Part Two:** Intervals x5 Rounds :45 sec on, :15 sec off *Total:* 20 minutes	• :20 sec side plank on knees (Left) • :20 side on Right • :20 Plank hold on knees *Total work time:* 3:00-4:30 **Part Two:** • Knee push ups • Up Downs • Sumo air squats • Russian twists

7	**AMRAP 20** As many reps as possible in 20 minutes. Rest as needed.	• 4 Knee push-ups • 8 Walking lunges each leg (16 total) • 12 Bicycle crunches
8	**EMOM 20-30** Each minute is a different movement. Build in transition to the next movement after 45 or 50 seconds.	**20 MIN** • Jumping Jacks • Tricep dips • Air Squats • Hollow Hold Pulses • Chair Step-ups
9	**TABATA x4** Do one movement for each Tabata round. (8 intervals in a row for each move) Rest one minute between each movement.	• Starburst Stands • Mountain climbers • Crunches • Table Pull ups *Total work time:* 16 minutes

10	**4 ROUNDS FOR TIME** Rest as needed.	• 20 Reverse Lunges • 10 Push ups • 10 Good Mornings • 20 Shoulder Taps
11	**DOUBLE UP INTERVALS** Do *two* working intervals for each movement before moving on to the next movement. *60 seconds of work each interval*	*Note:* Rest 60 sec after each interval *and* in between each movement at all levels. • Skater Steps • 100s: table top position • Air squats *Optional fourth movement:* knee plank hold
12	**Part One:** Five sets, rest 60 sec between sets (Do both moves before rest.) **Part Two:** **12 MIN AMRAP**	• 7 pike pushup • 3-5 knee push ups Rest 2-3 minutes, then: **Part Two:** • 12 Reverse lunges • 10 Step ups • 8 Up downs

16	**ALTERNATING TABATA** Alternate between the two movements for the first round and the other two movements in the second round. **Optional:** *Repeat one or both Tabata Rounds*	First Tabata Round: • Alt Toe Touches • Mountain Climbers Rest 1:00 Second Tabata Round: • Air Squats • Knee push ups
17	**Part One:** **EMOM 10** Min 1: 1st move Min 2: 2nd move **Part Two:** **6:00 Intervals x4 rounds:** Complete all movements then rest the remaining time of the six min. window.	• 8-10 Starbursts • 8-10 Push ups **Part Two:** • 300m brisk walk / 600m bike • 20 air squats • 30 crunches • 10 pushups
18	**FIVE ROUNDS FOR TIME** Rest as needed.	• 40 Jumping Jacks • 30 Lunges • 20 Sit ups • 10 Squats + press arms overhead • 5 Table pull ups

9

MID-RANGE LEVEL

"KICK IT UP A NOTCH" WORKOUTS ONLY

This chapter provides all the workouts from the "Kick It Up A Notch" level in one place. Some equipment will be needed.

1	EMOM 20 Minute 1: first movement Minute 2: second movement Minute 3: third movement Minute 4: fourth movement Minute 5: rest	• A-skips • Superman holds • Glute bridges • Bent over rows • Rest
2	**Descending & Ascending Ladder** 10-9-8-7-6-5-4-3-2-1 Run / row / bike 1-2-3-4-5-6-7-8-9-10	• Burpees • Toe Tap leg extensions • 300m run / 400m row / 500m bike (~90 seconds) *Use cardio as active rest or rest if needed
3	**AMRAP 15** As many reps as possible in 15 minutes. Rest as needed.	• 5 Knee push ups • 10 Banded air squats • 30 Alt. lunges, 15 each leg

4	**21-15-9** *Optional:* add a 200m jog/bike/row after finishing each number (all 21s, all 15s, and all 9s)	• Romanian Deadlift • Squat, then stand with toe raise, stretch arms overhead • Bent over row • Bench press
5	**Sprints X10** Choose running, rowing or biking. Stick with the same movement for all 10 rounds, giving max effort.	• 75m run / 125m row / 175m bike • Rest 1 minute • Repeat 9 times
6	**Part One:** 3 Rounds of: Side Planks & Plank holds **Part Two:** Intervals x5 Rounds :45 sec on, :15 sec off *Total:* 20 minutes	• :30 sec side plank on L • :30 side plank on R • :30 Front Plank hold *Total work time: 3:00-4:30* **Part Two:** • Push ups • Russian KBS • Sumo squats • Russian twists

7	**AMRAP 20** As many reps as possible in 20 minutes. Rest as needed.	• 4 Push-ups • 8 Suitcase lunges each leg (1 weight) • 16 Alt toe taps
8	**EMOM 20-30** Each minute is a different movement. Build in transition to the next movement after 45 or 50 seconds.	**25 MIN** • Penguin Hops • Tricep dips • Banded Squats • Hollow Holds • Box Step Ups
9	**TABATA x4** Do one movement for each Tabata round (8 intervals in a row for each move) *Total work time:* 16 minutes	• Starburst Jumps • Mountain climbers • Full Sit ups • Bent Over Row Rest one minute between each movement.

10	**4 ROUNDS FOR TIME** Rest as needed.	• 20 Jumping Lunges • 10 Push up burpees • 10 Romanian Deadlift • 20 Diagonal Planks
11	**DOUBLE UP INTERVALS** Do *two* working intervals for each movement before moving on to the next movement. *90 seconds of work each interval*	Rest 60 sec after each interval *and* in between each movement at all levels. • Skater Slides • 100s: legs extended • Banded Squats *Optional fourth movement: plank hold*
12	**Part One:** Five sets, rest 60 sec between sets (Do both moves before rest.) **Part Two: 12 MIN AMRAP**	• 8 strict press • 4-6 push ups Rest 2-3 minutes, then: **Part Two:** • 12 Jumping lunges • 10 Box jumps • 8 Burpees

13	**Part One:** 3 Rounds of: Side Planks & Plank holds **Part Two: AMRAP 18** As many reps as possible in 18 minutes.	• :30 sec side plank on L • :30 side plank on R • :30 Front Plank hold *Total work time: 3:00-4:30* **Part Two:** • 6 Push ups • 10 Thrusters • 150m run / 300m bike
14	**Ascending & Descending Ladder:** 20-18-16-14...2 Rest 2 minutes. 2-4-6-8-10...20	• Dumbbell deadlift • Toe Taps • KB / DB Swings
15	**AMRAP 18/21/24** Rest as needed. **Optional:** Add a 200m run/row or 400m bike after each round.	**21 MIN** • 75 Single Unders • 25 Air Squats • 10 Burpees • 5 Strict press

16	**ALTERNATING TABATA** Alternate between the two movements for the first round and the other two movements in the second round. **Optional:** *Repeat one or both Tabata Rounds*	First Tabata Round: • Alternating V-Ups • Mountain Climbers Rest 1:00 Second Tabata Round: • Jumping Squats • Push ups
17	**Part One:** **EMOM 10** Min 1: 1st move Min 2: 2nd move **Part Two:** **6:00 Intervals x4 rounds:** Complete all movements then *rest* the remaining time of the six min. window.	• 10-12 Alt Snatches • 10-12 Floor press **Part Two:** • 400m jog/row or 600m bike • 20 goblet squats • 20 sit ups • 10 burpees
18	**FIVE ROUNDS FOR TIME** Rest as needed.	• 40 Penguin Hops • 30 Jumping lunges • 20 Sit ups • 10 DB Thrusters • 5 Bent over row

10

HIGH-RANGE LEVEL

"TURBO BOOST ME" WORKOUTS ONLY

This chapter provides all the workouts from the "Turbo Boost Me" level in one place. Equipment will be needed.

1	**EMOM 20** Minute 1: first movement Minute 2: second movement Minute 3: third movement Minute 4: fourth movement Minute 5: rest	• Goblet March • Thrusters with DB • Glute bridges w/ DB over hips • Pull Ups • Rest
2	**Descending & Ascending Ladder** 10-9-8-7-6-5-4-3-2-1 Run / row / bike 1-2-3-4-5-6-7-8-9-10	• Pushup Burpees • V-Ups • 400m run / 500m row / 600m bike (~2 min) – Use cardio as active rest or rest if needed
3	**AMRAP 15** As many reps as possible in 15 minutes. Rest as needed.	• 5 Push ups • 10 Goblet squats • 30 Weighted alt. lunges, 15 each leg

4	**21-15-9** *Optional:* add a 200m jog/bike/row after finishing each number (all 21s, all 15s, and all 9s)	• Romanian Deadlift • Thrusters with DB • Pull Ups • Bench Press
5	**Sprints X10** Choose running, rowing or biking. Stick with the same movement for all 10 rounds, giving max effort.	• 100m run/ 150m row/ 200m bike • Rest 1 minute • Repeat 9 times
6	**Part One:** 3 Rounds of: Side Planks & Plank holds **Part Two:** Intervals x5 Rounds :45 sec on, :15 sec off *Total:* 20 minutes	• :30 sec side kneeling side plank w/ leg lift left side • :30 right side • :30 Front Plank hold *Total work time:* 3:00-4:30 **Part Two:** • Push ups • Full KBS • Sumo squats w/ high pull • Russian twists (weighted)

7	**AMRAP 20** As many reps as possible in 20 minutes. Rest as needed.	• 4 Push-ups • 4 Pike push-ups • 16 Walking suitcase lunges (2 weights) • 16 Alt V-ups
8	**EMOM 20-30** Each minute is a different movement. Build in transition to the next movement after 45 or 50 seconds.	**30 MIN** • Double Unders • Tricep dips • Goblet Squats • Hollow Rocks • Box Jumps
9	**TABATA x4** Do one movement for each Tabata round. Rest one minute between each movement. *Total work time:* 16 minutes	• Alternating Snatches • Mountain climbers • V-Ups • Pull Ups

10	**4 ROUNDS FOR TIME** Rest as needed.	• 20 Jumping Lunges • 10 Devils press • 10 Romanian Deadlift • 20 Plank Walks
11	**DOUBLE UP INTERVALS** Do *two* working intervals for each movement before moving on to the next movement. *120 seconds of work each interval*	Rest 60 sec after each interval *and* in between each movement at all levels. • Skater Slides • 100s: mix table top and extended • Banded / Goblet Squats • Plank Pull Throughs
12	**Part One:** Five sets, rest 60 sec between sets (Do both moves before rest.) **Part Two:** **12 MIN AMRAP**	• 7-9 seated press • 5-7 push ups Rest 2-3 minutes, then: **Part Two:** • 12 Reverse suitcase lunges • 10 Box jumps • 8 Burpees

13	**Part One:** 3 Rounds of: Side Planks & Plank holds **Part Two:** **AMRAP 18** As many reps as possible in 18 minutes.	• :30 sec side kneeling side plank w/ leg lift left side • :30 right side • :30 Front Plank hold *Total work time: 3:00-4:30* **Part Two:** • 8 Push ups • 12 Thrusters • 200m run / 400m bike
14	**Ascending & Descending Ladder:** 20-18-16-14…2 Rest 2 minutes. 2-4-6-8-10…20	• Dumbbell deadlift • Full sit ups • KB / DB Swings
15	**AMRAP 18/21/24** Rest as needed. **Optional**: Add a 200m run/row or 400m bike after each round.	**24 MIN** • 50 Double Unders • 25 Banded Squats • 10 Burpees • 5 Seated press

16	**ALTERNATING TABATA** Alternate between the two movements for the first round and the other two movements in the second round. **Optional:** *Repeat one or both Tabata Rounds*	First Tabata Round: • Double Leg V-Ups • Mountain Climbers Rest 1:00 Second Tabata Round: • Goblet Squats • Pike push ups
17	**Part One:** **EMOM 10** Min 1: 1st move Min 2: 2nd move **Part Two:** **6:00 Intervals x4 rounds:** Complete all movements then *rest* the remaining time of the six min. window.	• 12-14 Alt Snatches • 10-14 Bench press **Part Two:** • 500m run/row • 20 goblet squats • 30 sit ups • 10 burpees
18	**FIVE ROUNDS FOR TIME** Rest as needed.	• 40 Double Unders • 30 Suitcase lunges • 20 Alt V-Ups • 10 DB Thrusters • 5 Pull ups

11

MOVING ON

W oohoo! You've finished the workouts! (Or maybe you're just thinking ahead to what to do once you have - good job on that also.) Once you've completed the workouts in this book, it's a great time to take your fitness journey into your own hands. Here are several next steps to consider:

1. **Create your own workouts.** Use the movements and styles you've learned to design your own HIIT workouts. Mix and match exercises to keep your routines fresh and challenging. For example, combine strength moves like squats and push-ups with cardio bursts like burpees or high knees.

2. **Cycle through previous workouts.** Revisit the workouts from the guide you just completed. If you did all the workouts at one level, try them

again at a different one. Look back to your fitness log. Use the notes you took to modify the intensity or duration, or even challenge yourself by adding an extra round or reducing rest times.

3. **Set new goals**. Consider what you want to achieve next. Whether it's improving endurance, building strength, or mastering specific movements, setting new goals can help keep you motivated.

4. **Experiment with different formats**. Use some of the workouts provided that were in one style (like EMOM), and switch them up into an ascending ladder, or certain rounds for time. This variety can keep your training exciting and effective.

5. **Try new equipment.** If you have access to additional equipment like resistance bands, kettlebells, or stability balls, incorporate them into your workouts for added challenge and versatility.

6. **Join a community**. Consider joining a fitness community or group for support, motivation, and accountability. Sharing your progress and workouts with others can be incredibly inspiring for everyone involved.

7. **Listen to your body**: Remember to pay attention to how your body feels and adjust your workouts accordingly. It's important to include

rest days, mobility work, and active recovery to prevent burnout and injury.

By taking these steps, you can maintain your fitness momentum and continue to challenge yourself in exciting new ways.

RESOURCES

BOOKS

Amen, D. (2022). You, Happier. Tyndale.

Lyon, G. (2023). *Forever Strong.* Atria Books.

Mosconi, L. (2020). *The XX Brain.* Allen & Unwin.

Thurlow, C. (2022). *Intermittent Fasting Transformation.* Avery.

YOUTUBE SITES

Atlantic Physical Therapy Center. (2021, Jan 18). *Lizard Pose for hips.* YouTube. https://youtu.be/jXk5dquBT6 w?si=NmBY1rc-iCvC_QPx

Atomic Athlete. (2020, May 5). *Star Burst.* YouTube. https://youtu.be/F6oPyLjGWAQ?si=bDwx-naGCW2J1jKeo

Chari Hawkins. (2023, Mar 20). *A-Skip: The Rhythm of Running Drills.* YouTube. https://youtu.be/O9wh-huxbxU?si=2ENO_IriBFDv5p2t

CrossFit. (2015, Jan 1). *The Air Squat.* YouTube. https://youtu.be/C_VtOYc6j5c?si=KvYJwTVuH-CA0NkXl

CrossFit. (2019, Aug 23). *The Box Jump.* YouTube. https://youtu.be/NBY9-kTuHEk?si=Zd55Qs-rNSj9P2El

CrossFit. (2019, Dec 12). *The Box Step-Up.* YouTube. https://youtu.be/5qjqD-HOUh-A?si=1tBYEdL3z309xE–

CrossFit. (2019, Aug 10). *The Burpee.* YouTube. https://youtu.be/auBLPXO8Fww?si=Bi-zOHloUmlhYclFU

CrossFit. (2015, Aug 19). *The Double-under.* YouTube. https://youtu.be/-tF3hUsPZAI?si=T9DMZzNSJZV3ff5k

CrossFit. (2019, Nov 10). *The Dumbbell Deadlift.* YouTube. https://youtu.be/JNpUNR-PQkAk?si=Jm0SHo3pNaiA6iFS

CrossFit. (2016, Dec 5). *The Dumbbell Power Snatch.* YouTube. https://youtu.be/9520DJiFmvE?si=7QuqHP-PyIrajMrPv

CrossFit. (2020, Mar 23). *The Dumbbell Press.* YouTube. https://youtu.be/AqzDJHxyn-wo?si=dEIdaNBLWxkUegET

CrossFit. (2020, Mar 23). *The Dumbbell Push Press.* YouTube. https://youtu.be/4tCaD42ghlc?si=suMTS-Gtil8HXfum9

CrossFit. (2016, Oct 12). *The Dumbbell Swing.* YouTube. https://youtu.be/uB-fq0HqGK0?si=VmpgTRg-PT1Akm0H7

CrossFit. (2019, Sep 19). *The Dumb-bell Thruster.* YouTube. https://youtu.be/u3wKkZ-jE8QM?si=1_k8yhYiH2FhefGp

CrossFit. (2017, Jan 4). *The Hollow Rock.* YouTube. https://youtu.be/p7j02V1fIzU?si=g0cE0sFW-cD3cizew

CrossFit. (2019, Oct 5). *The Kettle-bell Swing.* YouTube. https://youtu.be/mKDIu-UbH94Q?si=h32hz_GR8U5lnenr

CrossFit. (2019, Feb 11). *The Push-Up.* YouTube. https://youtu.be/0pkjOk0EiAk?si=1GsBJ2VFoUYN-twXu

CrossFit. (2019, Feb 1). *The Strict Pull Up.* YouTube. https://youtu.be/HRV5YKKaeVw?si=ha-Jkt8H9qyxOD2sp

CrossFit. (2015, May 25). *The Walking Lunge.* YouTube. https://youtu.be/L8fvypPrzzs?si=MgF6Ahn zKQdaBT7d

CrossFit. (2019, Jul 11). *The V-Up.* YouTube. https://youtu.be/7UVgs18Y1P4?si=8Fgb7TTA6OC9qZ80

CrossFit CDA. (2020, Mar 29). *Body Weight Good Mornings.* YouTube. https://youtu.be/nczH_7m1TnI?si=OUdsWECDC7j2vFOi

CSIRO Total Wellbeing Diet. (2018, Oct 15) *Plank hold.* YouTube. https://youtu.be/J3QKdw79lNw?si=I8b SVVjq7yBFyXXC

CSIRO Total Wellbeing Diet. (2018, Oct 25) *Wall push up.* YouTube. https://youtu.be/-KVhapnEtuk?si=ALHz qcMUidN4QbWi

Dan Sroda Nutrition. (2016, Jul 7) *Table pull ups.* YouTube. https://youtu.be/woGSKA2tPrY?si=VNhsDE dfGkI9zTsu

David Diley. (2023, Sep 4). *Best Dumbbell Bench Press Tutorial Ever Made.* YouTube. https://youtu.be/1V3vp-caxRYQ?si=JVMCEtdIiMCItJGk

Dr. Chris || Pelvic Floor Physical Therapist. (2019, Feb 1). *Kneeling Side Plank + Leg Lift.* YouTube. https://yo utu.be/MdjSIC7SgoE?si=Z3fEZ8eUW-sZ819E

Functional Bodybuilding. (2019, Sep 29) *Devil Press.* YouTube. https://youtu.be/zlqEtAUds-I?si=VwcWqJml xrB3wilE

Functional Bodybuilding. (2018, Jun 20) *Dumbbell Romanian Deadlift.* YouTube. https://youtu.be/UsOjCcxS-JaI?si=zTet6UxCMfh640lT

Functional Bodybuilding. (2019, Feb 16) *Plank DB Pull Through.* YouTube. https://youtu.be/Zko5x2SoQmo?si=n-KQHJUUrMYCMc9a

Functional Bodybuilding. (2020, Feb 29) *Plank Shoulder Taps.* YouTube. https://youtu.be/C6At19Q9i2Q?si=YQG0wIJTALj_4WDX

Get Healthy U - with Chris Freytag. (2016, Sep 23). *How to do Full Sit Ups Properly (For Best Results!)* https://youtu.be/Q15ClFuxfeM?si=ZO4qyLnzII6hVft_

Get Healthy U - with Chris Freytag. (2019, Jan 29). *How to do Skaters.* YouTube. https://youtu.be/Jx2KXGbQkYM?si=_nYZBhoyhND4rA8U

Kettlebell Athletes. (2023, Nov. 29). *Kettlebell Goblet March.* YouTube. https://youtu.be/aAFF0WrHnfU?si=Q-kP_hiJDrRO8yZC

KINETICOACH The Travel Trainer. (2017, Feb 19). *Penguin Jumps.* YouTube. https://youtu.be/XA5SbAIRNFg?si=NEoTyGJw-dBDGzUW

Leap Fitness. (2020, Sep. 29) *How to Do: Abdominal Crunches.* YouTube. https://youtu.be/RUNrHkbP4Pc?si=JgaNoCjGSRzEE7Fj

Leap Fitness. (2020, Oct. 19) *How to Do: Diagonal Plank.*

YouTube. https://youtu.be/OGfFtF-dhrk?si=Jyr2ERSu0MhTsQ2V

Leap Fitness. (2020, Sep. 29) *How to Do: Jumping Jacks.* YouTube. https://youtu.be/2W4ZNSwoW_4?si=QH5RBndmptN1ZPVA

Leap Fitness. (2020, Oct. 16) *How to Do: Inchworms.* YouTube. https://youtu.be/ZY2ji_Ho0dA?si=Au_FNXkaa2uzdnN4

Leap Fitness. (2020, Oct. 13) *How to Do: Knee Push-Ups.* YouTube. https://youtu.be/jWxv-ty2KROs?si=GOsFZGyg4zEtrtQ0

Leap Fitness. (2020, Oct. 16) *How to Do: Lateral Plank Walk.* YouTube. https://youtu.be/yCVyaX-RjLM?si=Fdx-qLLeUStVPYCG5

Leap Fitness. (2020, Sep 29) *How to Do: Side Plank.* YouTube. https://youtu.be/2W96p2PI-oPg?si=UsdaD4j2QhhGT8XU

LiveStrong.com (2009, Jul 1) *How to Do Triceps Bench Dips.* YouTube. https://youtu.be/0326dy_-CzM?si=e_7Z9tHl2-BAhtns

LiveStrongWoman. (2014, Jun 18) *Mountain Climbers.* YouTube. https://youtu.be/zT-9L3CEcmk?si=XWFQANfTnIMk05G0

LiveStrongWoman. (2014, Apr 23) *Russian Twist*. YouTube. https://youtu.be/JyUqwkVpsi8?si=6ZDrkoD5 yfmf0L17

LiveStrongWoman. (2014, Apr 23) *Toe Tap*. YouTube. https://youtu.be/Ml2xTP45jVQ?si=4MR-rBOBfpgDN4RO9

Marcus Filly. (2018, Apr 6) *Dumbbell Bent Over Row*. Y o u T u b e . https://youtu.be/VP_f9V854og?si=_PWvGM8j7lrDo38Z

National Academy of Sports Medicine. (2018, Nov 19). How do to a Pike Push-Up. YouTube. https://youtu.be/ XckEEwa1BPI?si=ZJ-mFAD0xzBN9ctF

NCFIT. (2020, Feb 5). *Bootstrappers*. https://youtu.be/-SAna4vOJhA?si=14VCZ8vtgy-WuHb6q

Opex Fitness. (2021, Mar 8). *Dumbbell High Pull*. YouTube. https://youtu.be/o0KJD3Xn3fc?si=aFWfcak CL-G67gJQ

Opex Fitness. (2021, Jan 21). *Dumbbell Sumo Squat*. YouTube. https://youtu.be/vBA3vy-OxJv0?si=QAFvU_QOvfdoyiHd

Painscale. (2022, Oct 29) *Leg Extension–Core Strength–Wellness–Chronic Pain Relief–PainScale*. YouTube. https://www.painscale.com/arti-cle/core-strength-leg-extension

Pivot Cycles. (2021, Jan 20) P21E: Suitcase Lunge Demo. YouTube. https://youtu.be/KOLD4DlhJ64?si=9vTdAE-flar6z_-dh

Power Pilates. (2018, Aug 7). *How to do The Hundred in Pilates.* YouTube. https://youtu.be/_ddZR-BGG6p0?si=sJfho9orLYZBtbzK

PureGym. (2018, Jan 26). *How To Do A Glute Bridge.* YouTube. https://youtu.be/tqp5XQPp-TxY?si=VmtXwMgUoVyYgiNS

PureGym. (2018, Jan 16). *How To Reverse Lunge.* YouTube. https://youtu.be/xrPteyQL-GAo?si=BNcNOY3r5f__JuEn -

Rec Gym Kirrawee. (2020, Apr 18) *Russian Kettlebell Swing (RKBS) -CrossFit Movement Library.* YouTube. https://youtu.be/_vtp1QiJjeY?si=cP7AWswL6lI6I0zb

Rec Gym Kirrawee. (2020, Apr 7) *Up Downs -CrossFit Movement Library.* YouTube. https://youtu.be/4NRFUKgNhs8?si=K_SL8P_o2xXR0Goo

Sports Performance Physical Therapy. (2108, Oct 19). *Deep Lunge Thoracic Rotation.* YouTube. https://youtu.be/BxLkf1V0M94?si=PUYO4ujScbFNzh5T

St. Elizabeth Healthcare. (2021, Oct 5). *ACL Injury Prevention Program: Plyometrics - Jumping Lunges.* YouTube. https://youtu.be/I4mIS7p6EfU?si=L6AhFyPcqF0bvFya

The Fit Ninja. (2015, Jul 5) *Push-up with chair modified.* YouTube. https://youtu.be/kJ5CpP_Vjdo?si=F-FXKx5zgsn7CBSR

XHIT Daily. (2102, Sep 24). *Exercise Tutorial - Superman.* YouTube. https://youtu.be/z6PJMT2y8GQ?si=7Gzl-hoZGILPGmh_z

ARTICLES

Verywellfit.com. (2023, May 26). *How to Do a Bicycle Crunch: Fitness Tips, Variations, and Common Mistakes* https://www.verywellfit.com/bicycle-crunch-exercise-3120058

National Safety Council Injury Council. (2023) *All Leading Causes of Death.* https://injuryfacts.nsc.org/all-injuries/deaths-by-demographics/all-leading-causes-of-death/?utm_source=google_search&utm_medium=cpc&utm_campaign=injury_facts_gps&utm_content=if&gad_source=1&gclid=CjwKCAjw0t63BhAUEiwA5xP54RW-54q0aDwe43VRj1WdjX8SJX7oje-jxvHl-NaSoee2zzT59EVkUvhoCqXsQAvD_BwE

ABOUT THE AUTHOR

After 19 years of public school teaching, Elisa Pool left her career, her CrossFit gym, and her house in Oregon so she could travel the world with her husband and two young kids. After two years of nomadic life, they settled in Florida, where she's passionate about helping other mamas love themselves in word and action so that their children learn to do the same.

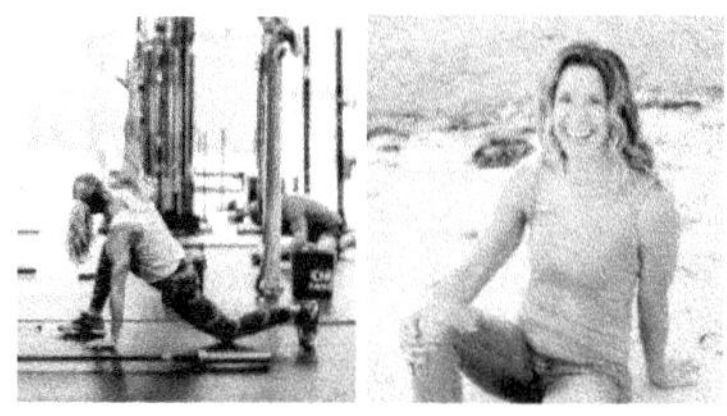

Muscles at work vs. muscles at rest. You won't bulk up, you'll tone up!

Photo Credit (in gym): Harrison Clark Photography

Photo Credit (on beach): Jess Veguez Photography

To contact the author:

Instagram: https://instagram.com/elisapool_wellness?igshid=OGQ5ZDc2ODk2ZA%3D%3D&utm_source=qr

Website: www.elisapoolwellness.com

Email: elisapoolwellness@gmail.com

www.ingramcontent.com/pod-product-compliance
Lightning Source LLC
Chambersburg PA
CBHW050811250726

48653CB00006B/2167